U0311970

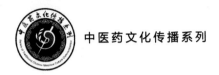

中医药文化传播系列

中医药文化概览

主 编◎毛国强 李兰兰 谭秀敏

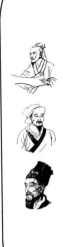

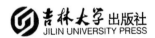

吉林大学出版社
JILIN UNIVERSITY PRESS

图书在版编目（CIP）数据

中医药文化概览 / 毛国强，李兰兰，谭秀敏主编. —长春：
吉林大学出版社，2019.4
ISBN 978-7-5692-4618-6

Ⅰ. ①中… Ⅱ. ①毛… ②李… ③谭… Ⅲ. ①中国医
药学－文化 Ⅳ. ①R2-05

中国版本图书馆CIP数据核字（2019）第071431号

书　　名	中医药文化概览	
	ZHONG-YIYAO WENHUA GAILAN	
作　　者	毛国强　李兰兰　谭秀敏　主编	
策划编辑	刘明明	
责任编辑	李欣欣	
责任校对	赵　莹	
装帧设计	中尚图	
出版发行	吉林大学出版社	
社　　址	长春市人民大街4059号	
邮政编码	130021	
发行电话	0431-89580028/29/21	
网　　址	http://www.jlup.com.cn	
电子邮箱	jdcbs@jlu.edu.cn	
印　　刷	河北盛世彩捷印刷有限公司	
开　　本	880mm×1230mm　1/32	
印　　张	5.25	
字　　数	65千字	
版　　次	2019年4月　第1版	
印　　次	2019年4月　第1次	
书　　号	ISBN 978-7-5692-4618-6	
定　　价	39.80元	

本书编委会成员

主　编：毛国强　李兰兰　谭秀敏

副主编：张　瑾　屠金莉　李　鹏　张　坚

编　委：段懿洲　耿晓娟　刘　佳　朱媛媛

（按拼音顺序排列）

总　序

中医药学源远流长,它凝聚了中华民族宇宙观、生命观、人生观的精华,同时也吸收了其他学科的知识成果。几千年来,硕果累累,名医辈出,一直守护着中华儿女的身心健康。中医药的价值不仅体现在精深的医学知识,还体现在丰厚的文化内涵。中医药文化具有强大的生命力和持续的创造力,是理解和传承中华优秀传统文化的重要抓手。

《中华人民共和国中医药法》的颁布、国务院发表《中国的中医药》白皮书,标志着中医药发展上升为国家战略,中医药事业进入新的历史发展时期。习近平总书记多次对中医药给予高度评价,他在给中国中医科学院60周年院庆的贺信中指出"中医药学凝聚着深邃的哲学智慧和中华民族几千年的健康养生理念及其实践经验，是中国古代科学的瑰宝，也是打开中华文明宝库的钥匙。深入研究和科学总结中医药学对丰富世界医学事业、推进生命科学研究具有积极意义"，同时希望广大中医药工作者"切实把中医药这一祖先留给我们的宝贵财富继承好、发展好、利用好，在建设健康中国、实现中国梦的伟大征程中谱写新的篇章"。2017年1月，中共中央办公厅、国务院办公厅印发了《关于实施中华优秀传统文化传承发展工程的意见》。中医药文化是中华优秀传统文化的重要组成部分，我们要通过多种形式向广大青少年传授基本的中医药文化知识，使他们了解中医药在日常生活、传统习俗、文学艺术等方方面面的文化蕴含，在他们心中播撒下热爱中医药文化的种子。

可喜的是，在天津市卫生健康委、天津市中医药管理局的高度重视下和大力支持下，2017和2018两年多时间里，天津中医药大学获得多个中医药文化研究方面的立项。其中，"中医药文化进校园"项目组负责人毛国强教授带领项目组成员，在开展中医药文化传播研究的同时,还开拓思路深入全市近20多所中小学试点校,开展了多项中医文化推广活动,包括中医药文化知识宣讲、中医保健讲座、中药囊制作,并组织大中小学生参观百年老字号中药厂,参加中医药文化主题夏令营、中医药主题诗词音乐朗诵会等,将中医药的知识传授与文化传承与传播活动很好地融合在一起。项目开展的两年时间里,全市数千名中小学生参与其中,许多学生表现出对中医药文化浓厚的兴趣,各种活动也在社会上引起较好的反响。为了满足青少年进一步了解中医药知识的需求,项目组组织邀请相关专家多次研讨,以天津中医药大学相关专业教师为主,在广泛吸纳了中小学教育专家、师生意见建议基础上,编写了《中医药文化精选读本》(小学版和中学版)。其中小学版读本立足小学生阅读特点,通过一个个小故事,辅以卡通漫画形象,讲述故事里蕴含的中医药文化知识以及浅显易懂的中医文化哲理,图文并茂,形象传神。在不增加孩子们负担的情况下,激发他们对中医药知识的好奇心和求知欲。中学版读本遵循中学生的认知规律,以通俗的科普小故事为载体,通过"识人体,解中医""读课本,学中药""观生活,明中医""体民俗,感中医""读名篇,叙中医"等五个章节传递中医药文化知识,化繁为简,深入浅出,培养中学生对于中医药文化的感知与热爱。作为此书的总主编,我曾多次参加这套读本的编写会议,编写组先后6次邀请全国及天津市各方面专家召开研讨论证、评审会,对读本构架、内容设计广泛征询意见,历时两年对文字内容、配图形式、板式设计等进行10多次修改、完善,精心组织、精细打磨、精益求精,力求既科学严谨通俗、又可读好看。相信,这套面向青少年的中医药文化读本会对他们了解中医药文化起到帮助作用,也会培养更多对中医药文化感兴趣的未来"中医药人"。

除了这两册面向青少年的读本以外,首批"中医药文化传播系列"中,面向中老年读者的《中医名家谈节气养生与文化》是在《中老年时报》颐寿专栏刊稿的基础上扩展而成,倾注了许多中医大家名家的心血。书中有对三位中国工程院院士、九位国医大师、十多位名中医的访谈，他们用通俗易懂的话语、生动形象的表述，为读者悉心讲授节气养生的要诀。如此多的大家、名家为老百姓普及中医养生、健康常识，在全国中医科普类书籍中是开先河的。除养生宝典外，编著者十分用心，还汇集了与节气有关的民俗、谚语、古诗词等深厚的节气文化内涵，相信读者定会开卷有益，受益匪浅。

中医药文化不仅是我国的优秀传统文化，还是全人类的精神财富。新形势下，我们应该讲好中医的"中国故事"，做好中医药文化国际传播这篇大文章。本套书中有两本以外国留学生和来华工作、旅行者为主要受众对象的书也同样值得关注。《中医药文化概览》为全英文读本，以中医零基础的外国人士为目标读者，面向来华工作、学习、生活、旅游并对中医药文化感兴趣的外国朋友。《读故事，识本草——中药入门读本》则是双语读本，目标读者是对中药感兴趣的外国人，及来华读书的留学生。该书介绍了五十种常见常用的中药，以及这些中药背后的有趣故事，还介绍了药材在食品、养生、化妆品、园林绿化等方面的利用价值。

作为在全国有影响力的中医药类高校，天津中医药大学在传承和发展中医药文化上责无旁贷。特别是在贯彻全国教育大会精神、建设国家"双一流"高校的契机下，文化传承与创新板块成为建设的一个重要内容。而文化的传承与活力需要动态的传播来体现，平台和载体的建设尤为重要。2017年，我校成立了中医药文化研究与传播中心，成立仅一年就成果颇丰，2018年即升级为天津市级机构，由天津市卫健委与我校共建。该中心落户在文化与健康传播学院，它们发挥人文学院优势，联合中医学院、中药学院及社会力量，不仅开展了10多项中医文化研究，还组织了形式多样的中医药文化主题大众传播活动。这一套书即是其中的成果之一。

我由衷希望这套书在传承和弘扬中医药文化方面发挥积极作用，成为国人乃至全世界了解和学习中医药文化的好帮手。

这套书的编写和出版，得到了众多中医药人、社会各界的帮助和支持。参与编写工作的专家、老师、同学们十分投入和认真，圆满地完成了预定任务。

尤其令我感动的是，德高望重，才艺双馨，在海内外享有盛誉，已经94岁高龄的古典诗词大家叶嘉莹先生，欣然为《中医名家谈节气养生与文化》一书撰写推介感言。在此，一并表示深深的敬意和衷心感谢。

中医药文化要从中国走向世界，要以传统面向未来。任重而道远，让我们一起努力！

中国工程院院士
天津中医药大学校长

2019年5月于天津团泊湖畔

张伯礼 中国工程院院士，全国名中医，中医内科学专家，天津中医药大学校长，国务院政府特殊津贴专家，国家有突出贡献中青年专家；国家"重大新药创制"重大专项技术副总师，国务院医政咨询专家委员会委员，教育部医学教育专家委员会副主任；参加国家中医药现代化顶层设计；参加起草了《中医现代化科技发展战略》《中药现代化发展纲要》等文件；作为全国人大代表提出《发展中医药健康服务业规划》等数十项议案和建议；提出并推动了《中医药法》颁布实施。

前　言

　　中医药学是中华民族的一张重要文化名片,具有神奇的凝聚力和无形的吸引力。其具有完整的理论体系和确切的临床疗效,在中国的医疗卫生保健体系中发挥着不可替代的重要作用,在世界上也得到了广泛应用,为提高世界各国人民的健康水平做出了贡献。

　　如今,中医药已传播到全球183个国家和地区,有86个国家政府与中国签订了有关中医药的合作协议,中国在国外建立了17个中医药中心,中国制定了一批国际中医药标准,建立了一批中医药"走出去"的合作基地。与此同时,中医药文化也吸引了世人的目光。越来越多的外国人士开始关注中医,喜欢中医。由于中西方文化的差异，理解中医药文化对外国人士来说比较困难。此书为纯英文读本，以中医零基础的外国人士为目标读者，主要面向来华工作、学习、生活、旅游并对中医药文化感兴趣的外国人。在一位来自中医世家名为东东的11岁中国小男孩的引领下，从介绍中医药基本知识入手，介绍了中医和西医的不同、中医治疗方法和中医院看病的体验等；和读者分享了四位中国古代著名医家的故事。通过东东亲身经历的几个小故事，说明了中医药的药食同源；以庖丁解牛和范进中举的故事分别引出中医养生的本质和常见养生方法，以及几种可以缓解疲劳的简单自我按摩手法。为了提高读本的可读性，本书配有大量的图片，其中很多插图是连环画风格，具有丰富的中国文化内涵。

此书作为天津市中医药文化研究与传播中心、天津中医药大学文化与健康传播学院策划、组织的"中医药文化传播系列"，得到了中医药文化传播中心荣誉主任、中国工程院院士、天津中医药大学校长张伯礼教授的大力支持。天津市卫生健康委员会、天津市中医药管理局中医处相关领导也对此书给予了支持和帮助，在此一并表示感谢。

　　因为水平有限，编写过程中难免会出现一些疏漏和不足之处，恳请各位专家、学者、同行和读者朋友们给予批评指正，并提出宝贵的意见和建议。

编　者

Preface

Traditional Chinese medicine culture, an important cultural card of China, radiates magical cohesion and attraction. Traditional Chinese medicine (TCM) has a complete theoretical system and curative effect. It not only plays an irreplaceable role in China's medical and health care system, but also is widely applied in the world, making contributions to the improvement of the health of the people in the world.

At present, Chinese medicine has been put in use in 183 countries and regions, passed to the people of the world. Cooperative protocols have been signed on Chinese medicine between 86 countries and China. China has founded 17 traditional Chinese medicine centres abroad. While going out, TCM culture has also attracted the attention of the world. More and more foreigners are paying attention to Chinese medicine and like it. However, due to the differences between Chinese and Western cultures, understanding Chinese medicine culture is more difficult for foreigners. This is an English book only for foreigners who don't learn TCM but work, study, live or travel in China and are interested in TCM. Under the guidance of an 11-year-old boy named Dongdong from a family of TCM, this book first introduces the basic knowledge of TCM. Starting with what TCM is, it briefly introduces the differences between TCM and Western medicine, the treatment methods of TCM and the experience of seeing a doctor in a hospital of TCM. Then four famous ancient doctors are introduced and four interesting stories are shared. Several events happening to Dongdong illustrate that food can be used as both food and medicine in TCM. Subsequently, the stories of *A Butcher Dismembering an Ox* and *Fan Jin Passing Civil Exam* are respectively introduced to show the essence of health preservation and several common methods in health preservation. Finally some simple self-massage techniques which can be used to relieve fatigue and treat insomnia are also introduced. In order to help readers understand it better, the book has a large number of pictures, many of which are of comic style with rich Chinese cultural connotations.

As one of the series of books about TCM culture planned and organized by Tianjin TCM Culture Research and Communication Center and College of Culture and Health Communication of Tianjin University of TCM, this book has received strong support from Professor Zhang Boli, honorary director of Tianjin TCM Culture Research and Communication

Center, academician of the Chinese Academy of Engineering and president of Tianjin University of TCM. Relevant leaders from Tianjin Municipal Health Committee, Department of Chinese Medicine, Tianjin Administration of TCM also gave much financial support and help to this book. We are deeply grateful to all of them.

However, the book might be imperfect due to the limited ability of the writers. Experts, scholars, peers and readers are welcome to give criticism and corrections, and provide valuable comments and suggestions.

Contents

1

Part Two

Great Physicians in Ancient China

Part Three

Stories in the History of TCM

Part Six

The Internationalization of TCM

Part One

Something You Need to Know about TCM

Hi! So glad you open this booklet and give me a chance to meet you. My name is Dongdong ("Dong" means "east" in Chinese). I am eleven years old and I was born in a family of traditional Chinese medicine (TCM). My grandfather and my parents are all TCM doctors. I am proud of my family. At the 2016 Summer Olympics, you might have seen athletes with purple circles on their skin from cupping. Or maybe you know someone who has herbal tea for colds. More and more people use practices like these from TCM to fight disease and prevent disease. Child as I am, I know a lot about TCM, and I can't wait to share with you.

In this part, let's find answers to the following four questions.

What is TCM?

How does TCM differ from Western medicine?

What are the ways of treatment in TCM?

What is a visit to a TCM practitioner like?

Besides I'll share you some facts about TCM.

OK, I'll start with the first question.

1. What is TCM ?

TCM is a medical system that began its development in China about 5,000 years ago. To tell you the truth, it's hard to explain what TCM is in simple words. My grandfather always tells me "TCM is an indispensable part of the splendid Chinese culture" and it is based on some theories in Chinese philosophy. I don't know much about philosophy, but I do know ancient Chinese philosophers believed that our body interacted with all aspects of life and the environment. The aspects included the seasons, weather, time of day, our diet and emotional states. TCM sees the key to health as the harmonious and balanced functioning of body and spirit.

Does my explanation puzzle you? If you feel it complicated to understand, it's reasonable. TCM is based on some ancient beliefs in China. To help you better understand what it is, I'll introduce you some basic ideas. These beliefs include the following:

•TCM is based on a philosophy of balance with nature. The understanding of human body is based on the holistic understanding of the universe. The human body is a miniature version of the larger, surrounding universe. In other words, individuals are viewed as a part of the forces of nature.

•TCM believes a human's body is a self-regulating system. Internally, it regulates to achieve a balance between each part, but sometimes it needs some outside help (with the help of TCM) to achieve that balance.

•Qi, (pronounced chee), is also called

life energy or vital energy that flows through the body, and it performs multiple functions in maintaining health. Qi runs throughout our body, though it can't be directly measured, or even detected through any known means. TCM believes it does exist and it's always on the move and constantly changes. TCM practitioners see disease as the result of disruptions in the movement or the transformation of qi.

•Health is the result of balance between yin and yang. Yin and yang are two opposing yet complementary forces in all things, for example, female-male, dark-light and old-young. Everything in life has a little bit of its opposite, too. When you balance the yin and yang of qi, you feel healthy and well. If they're out of whack, you feel sick. Yin and yang are also used to describe the qualities of qi.

So far, are you still with me? I guess you may get a general understanding of TCM, but you still don't know what exactly it is. Don't worry. All you need to do is to remember TCM helps live in harmony with natural environment with the aim of keeping all aspects of a person including mind, body, and spirit, in a state of harmony and balance so that disease never has a chance to develop.

Now let's move on to the second question.

2. How does TCM differ from Western medicine?

In theory and practice, TCM is completely different from Western medicine, both in terms of considering how the human body works and how illness occurs and should be treated.

To make it clear, let's see a picture.

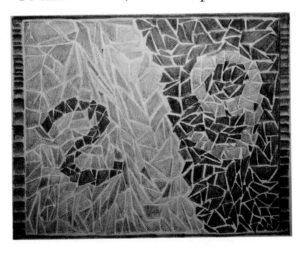

What do you see from the picture? For Western medicine this is a picture with small colorful dots. TCM finds there is a reversed letter "S" and a number "9". In fact, both medical systems deal with the same objective (human body). Their conclusion is different since the angle of view is different. Western medicine focuses on details while TCM concentrates on the whole.

The word "patient" has different meanings for Western medicine and TCM. From the perspective of Western medicine, a patient would be viewed as a basically healthy individual with a particular problem. In Chinese medicine, however, disease is not viewed as something that a patient has. It is an imbalance in the patient's being. Therefore, Western medicine focuses mainly on treating disease. But TCM looks at your entire well-being. Western medicine tends to view the body a lot like a car. It has different systems that need the right inputs and outputs. It's very concrete and logical, whereas TCM is based on balance, harmony, and energy. One of its guiding principles is to "dispel the bad and support the good". In addition to treating illness, TCM focuses on strengthening the body's defenses and enhancing its capacity for healing and maintaining health.

In TCM, treatment is not based only on the symptoms, but differentiation of syndromes. A patient goes to see a TCM doctor. When the doctor evaluates the syndrome, he or she considers not only the cause, mechanism, location, and nature of the disease, but also the confrontation between pathogenic factor and body resistance. Therefore, those with an identical disease may be treated in different ways, and on the other hand, different diseases may result in the same syndrome and are treated in similar ways. I know this is difficult to understand. Let me share you two examples. One day two patients with the same symptom of high fever and constipation went to see a famous TCM doctor. One was given herbal medicines to relax bowels. The other got medicines to induce perspiration. Surprisingly they were recovering. When asked, the doctor answered, "The same symptoms resulted from different causes. One patient suffered from exogenous pathogenic factors. The other was attacked by internal damp-heat. So they were treated differently. " The other day, two women patients with different symptoms went to the TCM doctor. One was diagnosed with gastroptosis (the abnormal downward displacement of the stomach), and the other was attacked by hysteroptosis (the abnormal downward displacement of the uterus). The doctor prescribed the same medicines. The patients were puzzled, and the doctor explained, "Your gastroptosis and her hysteroptosis are both caused by sinking of middle qi, so I used the same medicine to elevate it." Treatment based on syndrome differentiation, one of the characteristics of TCM, is the basic principle in TCM for understanding and treating diseases.

Many people believe the main difference between Chinese medicine and Western medicine is that Chinese medicine seeks to treat the body as a whole, while Western medicine focuses on the main problem area. Neither one is wholly right nor wholly wrong; instead they complement one another. I feel the same.

Do you know the ways of treatment in TCM? Have you ever tried any of them? In the following, let's focus on the third question.

3. What are the ways of treatment in TCM?

As well as giving a diagnosis, TCM also includes many treatments to help people stay healthy, including acupuncture, moxibustion (burning an herb above the skin to apply heat to acupoints), Chinese herbal medicine, tuina (Chinese therapeutic massage), qi gong (practices that combine specific movements or postures, coordinated breathing, and mental focus) and cupping.

Let me introduce them to you one by one.

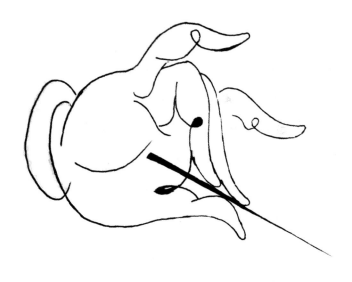

Acupuncture: Acupuncture is a technique in which practitioners stimulate specific points on the body—most often by inserting thin needles through the skin. I know you want to ask "Does acupuncture hurt?" Surprisingly, although needles are used in acupuncture, treatments are relatively pain-free. In fact, one of the most popular uses of acupuncture is to reduce chronic pain throughout the body in a natural way, and you don't need to worry about unwanted side effects.

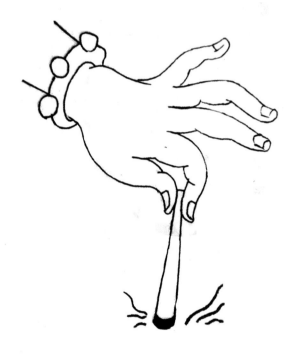

Moxibustion: A burning cigar-shaped *moxa* stick is usually made of herbs, which are called mugwort or wormwood. The stick is held near acupoints to stimulate them with heat and improve the flow of qi. It is used along with acupuncture and TCM practitioners may recommend it for improvement of general health as well as for cancer and treatment of chronic conditions such as arthritis and digestive disorders.

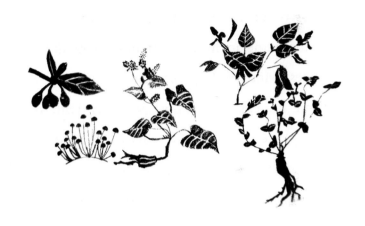

Chinese herbal medicine: In TCM, herbal medicine includes thousands of medicinal substances. Most of them are plants, but there are also some minerals and animal products. Different parts of plants, such as the leaves, roots, stems, flowers, and seeds, are used. In TCM, herbs are often combined in formulas and given as tea, capsules, liquid extracts, or powders.

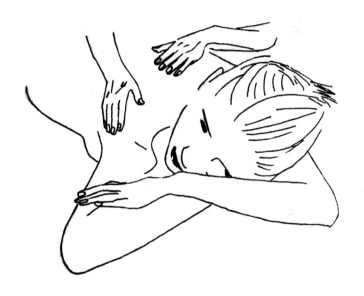

Tuina: Generally speaking, tuina is used in TCM to treat diseases with muscles. Practitioners may brush, knead, roll, press and rub the suffering body parts. For example, if you suffer from back pain, a practitioner may press and rub your back, and then use range of motion, traction, massage, with the stimulation of acupressure points.

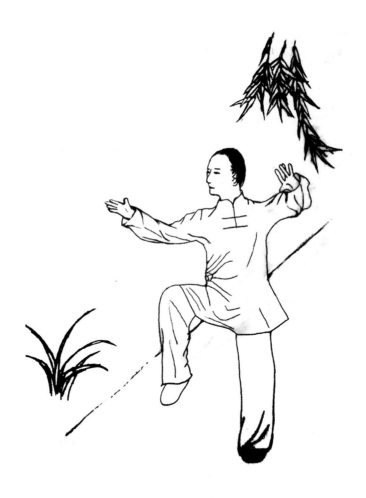

Qigong: Qigong has a history of over 5,000 years. It is a mind-body practice as well as an energetic form of movement. People practice it to enhance the flow of qi in body. By integrating posture, body movements, breathing and focused intention, qigong is designed to improve mental and physical health. Some experts believe that there are more than 3,000 different styles of qigong in existence today.

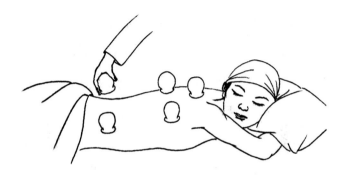

Cupping: This 2,500-year-old practice involves placing special cups filled with heated air on painful areas of the body. As the cups cool, the volume of air within them shrinks, creating suction on the skin that increases blood flow to the area. It is commonly used to ease aches and pains, relieve respiratory problems, lessen coughs and wheezing and improve circulation. Cupping can leave bruises that can take a week or more to fade. The mysterious dots on Michael Phelps at 2016 Rio Olympics were the result of cupping. Many athletes admit cupping saves them from a lot of pain.

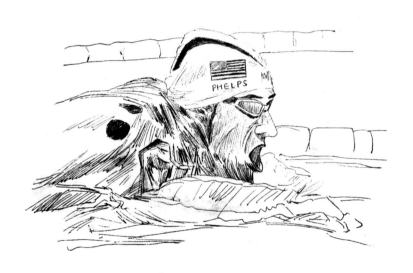

Do you think TCM is mysterious and magical? In fact, it is not so strange as you've imagined. If you don't believe me, you can go to a TCM practitioner to experience when you need to see a doctor. Let's try to find what to expect on a visit to a TCM practitioner.

4. What is a visit to a TCM practitioner like?

During your first visit, a TCM practitioner will make a detailed assessment of your overall health in order to identify any imbalance. The practitioner will use four methods of diagnosis (四诊 sizhen). These four methods include observation (望诊 wangzhen), auscultation and olfaction (闻诊 wenzhen), interrogation (问诊 wenzhen) and pulse feeling and palpation (切诊 qiezhen). The moment you walk in the clinic, the practitioner has begun the observation. He or she observes your complexion, the way you walk, the voice of your talking, the brightness of your hair etc. While you are seated, the doctor will exam your pulse of each arm with his index, middle and ring fingers. The rhythm, strength and volume of your pulse will be described with qualities like "floating, slippery, feeble, thready and quick". Each of the quality indicates certain disease pattern. Meanwhile, you will be asked to show your tongue to examine its shape, size, color and texture. Then the practitioner will ask you about your subjective sensations of temperature, such as "what do you habitually feel, hot or cold?" You'll also be asked about your sleep habits, the state of your appetite and digestion, and your thirst levels. If you report pain, the practitioner will ask what makes it better or worse. Then, a treatment plan will be customized for you to support the flow of qi in your body. This may include acupuncture, dietary advice, prescription of one or more herbal formulas or a combination of treatments.

Besides what I have told you above, below

are some facts about TCM to help you understand more about it.

4.1 TCM has clear branches.

TCM is not just about taking a patient's pulse and drinking herbal potions. It has clear branches, just as Western medicine does.

4.2 Most TCM drugs are acquired easily from plants.

Chinese people have used nature's power to keep healthy for a long time. For example, the most well-known TCM herbs are goji berries, ginger, and cinnamon. Goji berries can nourish liver and kidney, benefit essence and blood, therefore many people, especially middle-aged men, like to drink goji berry tea to preserve health.

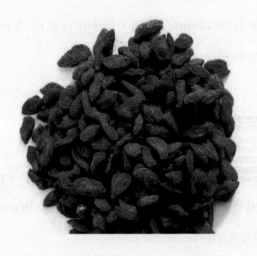

4.3 There's no fixed recipe in TCM.

The same medicinal materials with different ratios can have different effects. Some curative formula might become harmful due to improper ratios. The recipe of each prescription is adjusted based on the patient's physical condition. Therefore, without professional consultation, you can't just use herbal medicine or treatment because of little side effects.

4.4 TCM hospitals are not 100% traditional nowadays.

In China, if you find TCM doctors carry out a blood test, don't feel surprised. Nowadays, machines are also used in TCM hospitals to help doctors make a diagnosis. Normally, patients can choose whether to take Western medicine or herbal concoctions and other TCM treatments.

After my introduction, have you been attracted by TCM which has withstood the tests of time? As time goes on, we all believe it will be better and be more accepted by more people in the future.

More reading

If you want to know more about TCM, please refer to the following links.

1.Origins & History of Chinese Medicine

https://www.sacredlotus.com/go/foundations-chinese-medicine/get/origins-history-chinese-medicine

2. The Role of Taoist Spirituality in Chinese Medicine, Part One: The Gate of All Wonders

https://www.acupuncturetoday.com/mpacms/at/article.php?id=30308

Part Two

Great Physicians in Ancient China

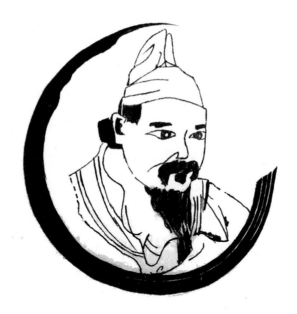

Hi! So glad to meet you again. In this part, I am going to introduce some great physicians in ancient China. In China's long history there were so many well-known doctors of TCM. Due to their outstanding contribution in this field, Chinese medical theory has been developed very well and still cherished today. Let us check out the most famous TCM physicians in ancient China and extend our salute to them.

In the following sections, you are to know something about four greatest ancient physicians: Hua Tuo, Zhang Zhongjing, Sun Simiao and Li Shizhen.

1. Hua Tuo

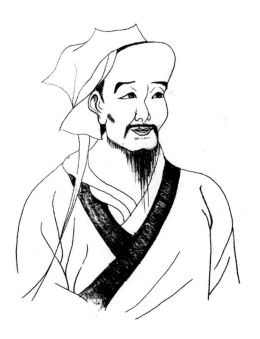

Hua Tuo was an ancient Chinese physician who lived during the late Han Dynasty and Three Kingdoms era. He was born in Haozhou, Anhui. Haozhou is one of the four cities of medicine in China.

Hua Tuo was born into a poor family. When he was seven years old, his father passed away, taking with him the only source of family income. Faced with financial hardship and poverty, Hua Tuo began to work in a local herbal pharmacy. While working there, he carefully observed the practice of medicine and pharmacy. Thus began his career as one of the best physicians.

Hua Tuo practiced medicine during the end of the Eastern Han and beginning of the Three Kingdoms, a period of time characterized by political instability with constant battles and turmoil. He sympathized with the common people whose lives were suppressed by the government and dedicated his entire life to helping them. Therefore, he was also known as "the physician of the people". He preferred to treat the common folks and repeatedly refused to accept offers of the position as the Supreme Physician in the Imperial Palace.

Hua Tuo is respected for being the first surgeon and inventor of Mafeisan (Numbing and Boiling Powder), an herbal formula used to stop patients feeling pain during a surgery in TCM. He believed that for diseases that could not be treated with acupuncture and herbs, the only solution was surgery to remove the cause. It is well-documented that Hua Tuo frequently performed surgery on various parts of the body by using Mafeisan for systemic anesthesia.

Despite his outstanding achievements, there were always more patients than Hua Tuo could possibly care for in his practice. Thus, he began to wonder why people were always sick and what would make them healthier. He believed that chronic illnesses were due, in part, to a lack of physical activity and proposed regular exercise as a remedy. As part of Hua Tuo's strong emphasis on the importance of physical activity, he developed Wuqinxi (Five Animal Frolics), an exercise that imitates the physical movement of tigers, deer, apes, bears and cranes.

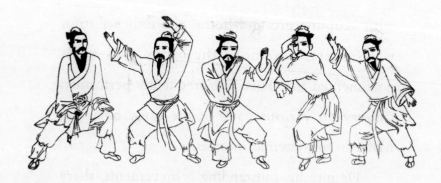

Of the stories told of Hua Tuo, one legend is that General Guan Yu, one of the great military heroes of the time who eventually became God of War, came to Hua Tuo because of an arrow wound in his arm that had become badly infected. The surgeon prepared to give his patient the usual anesthetic drink, but General Guan Yu laughed scornfully and called for a board and stones for a game of go. While Hua Tuo scraped the flesh and bone free of infection and repaired the wound, Guan Yu and one of his military companions proceeded calmly with their game.

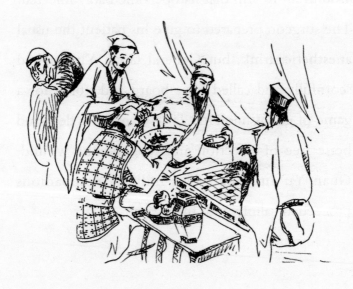

In his later years, Hua Tuo was called by the emperor of the Wei Kingdom, Cao Cao, to treat his "head wind" (presumably migraine headache) that had not responded to any of the treatments by many other physicians. By the insertion of just one needle, the chronic headache was alleviated. Cao was so impressed that he insisted on having Hua Tuo as his personal physician. However, Hua Tuo tactfully refused, claiming he needed to return home to attend to his sick wife.

Shortly after returning home, he was called again and subsequently forced by Cao to return to the Imperial Palace. Cao had another severe headache and wanted Hua Tuo to cure him and would not let him leave the Imperial Palace. Hua Tuo stated the headache was so severe that it could not be treated simply with herbs or acupuncture. The only cure would be to induce anesthesia and surgically open the head to remove the cause of the headache. Cao thought Hua Tuo was making an attempt to assassinate him and sentenced Hua Tuo to death.

While in prison, Hua Tuo compiled all of his clinical experience in writing and tried to give it to a prison guard for safe keeping. However, out of fear of Cao, the guard refused to do any favors or accept anything from Hua Tuo. In extreme anger and frustration, Hua Tuo burned his manuscripts, turning all his clinical knowledge to ashes. After Hua Tuo died, he was buried next to a flowing river of clear water—symbolizing he was cleared from all wrong-doing.

2. Zhang Zhongjing

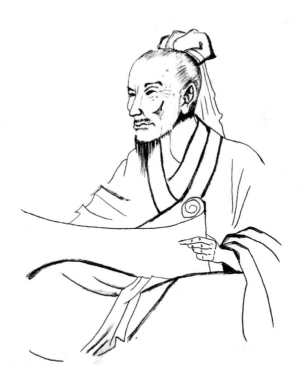

Zhang Zhongjing (A.D. 150—219), commonly known as Zhang Ji, was a famous physician from the Eastern Han Dynasty. He was known for his book *Shang Han Za Bing Lun* (《伤寒杂病论》 *Treatise on Cold Pathogenic and Miscellaneous Disease*), which was the most influential and impactful medical book in the development of Chinese medicine. It was also the first monumental work on clinical medical treatment in China. This book effectively developed and established the theoretical framework for Chinese medical diagnoses and treatment. His book is highly regarded by doctors of all ages, and he is admired as the Saint of Medicine.

Zhang Zhongjing was born in Nanyang, Henan Province. His home town was one of the four cities of medicine in China. While still a young man, Zhang Zhongjing took a special interest in medicine. In his time, many people were infected with febrile disease, as was his own family. He learned medicine by studying from Zhang Bozu, a fellow townsman, from other carefully—studied medicinal texts, and by accumulating prescriptions from around China.

When Zhang Zhongjing was a prefect of Changsha, disease prevailed in the country. As medicine was not very developed then, many people, especially the poor, turned to witchcraft when they were sick, only turned out to be cheated. Zhang Zhongjing was truly upset with what he observed. He hated the shamans, who brought death upon people for money.

Once he saw a woman suffering because of her illness. She was crying and laughing, obviously under some form of stimulation. Zhang Zhongjing took a closer look at the patient and pointed out that she was in fact suffering from internal heat in her blood chamber, which could be cured. He applied acupuncture to the patient, who healed after a few days.

One day, while Zhang Zhongjing was working as a physician, he saw a group of people gathered in front of a house. He went forward to examine the situation. A man was lying on the floor with a few women crying next to him. Zhang Zhongjing was told that the man had hanged himself because he was too poor to continue living. Zhang kept the man warm by covering him with a blanket. Then he asked two men to press on the man's chest. Zhang Zhongjing then exerted pressure with his palms on the man's abdomen and waist a few times. After a while, the man came around.

Zhang's masterpiece, *Shang Han Za Bing Lun*, was collected and organized later by physicians, notably Wang Shuhe from the Jin Dynasty and various court physicians during the Song Dynasty into two books, namely for the former, *Shanghan Lun* (《伤寒论》*Treatise on Cold Pathogenic Diseases*), which was mainly on a discourse on how to treat epidemic infectious diseases causing fevers prevalent during his era, and the latter, a highly influential doctrine *Jin Gui Yao Lue* (《金匮要略》*Synopsis of Golden Chamber*), a compendium of various clinical experiences which was regarded as a main discourse on internal diseases. These two texts have been heavily reconstructed several times up to the modern era.

3. Sun Simiao

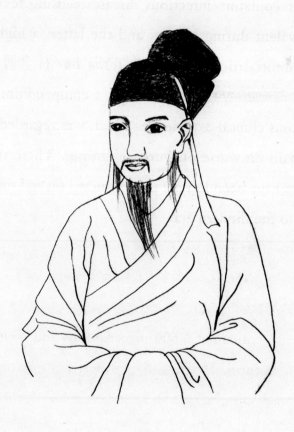

Sun Simiao (581—682) was the greatest doctor in the Tang Dynasty. When he was young, Sun Simiao was very intelligent but frequently suffered from diseases. He was well educated and read books of various schools, including medicine. Two emperors of the Tang dynasty invited him to work in the Imperial Court, but he refused to accept. All through his life, he lived in the mountains, practicing and studying medicine. He lived for over one hundred years and was worshiped as King of Medicine.

Sun Simiao wrote two books, *Qian Jin Yao Fang* (《千金要方》 *Golden Prescriptions*) and *Qian Jin Yi Fang* (《千金翼方》 *Supplement to Golden Prescriptions*), thirty volumes each. These two books contained 6,500 prescriptions and covered the aspects of life cultivation, acupuncture, moxibustion, medicines and other related fields. So *Qian Jin Yao Fang* was both a comprehensive book of medicine and an encyclopedia of medicine.

Qian Jin Yao Fang was different from other medical books in content arrangement. For instance, he put the part about prevention and treatment of women diseases during pregnancy and nursing of the newborn at the beginning of the first volume. Such an arrangement may indicate that Sun Simiao respected women or advocated the concept of protecting and caring life from birth.

Besides, Sun Simiao also discussed extensively that doctors should cultivate their mind. He said a doctor should be well learnt and hard working; regard patients as his relatives, avoid being self-proud and never slander other doctors. He wrote an article about the morality for doctors known as *Da Yi Jing Cheng* (《大医精诚》 *On the Absolute Sincerity of Great Physicians*) which was so great and important that was often called "the Chinese

Hippocratic Oath".

Sun Simiao died in A.D. 682. He is treated respectfully by later generations. People built temples, carved statues and built up public image for him. His books are widely printed and spread overseas, becoming important TCM works.

4. Li Shizhen

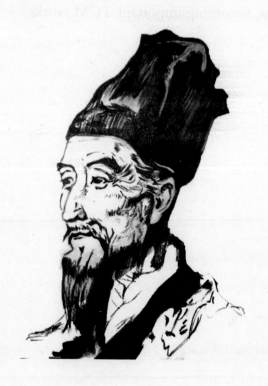

Li Shizhen (1518—1593) was a famous medical scholar who has sort of the same stature as Leonardo da Vinci in the West. He was born in Hubei in 1518 at a time of relative prosperity in the middle of the Ming dynasty.

He is mainly known for laboring for most of his life on medical treatises and for publishing a very long encyclopedia of natural medicine called *Ben Cao Gang Mu* (《本草纲目》 *Compendium of Materia Medica*). The text is highly detailed and organized, and it is the product of decades of study of rare books and medical texts. He added his own understanding derived from his own medical practice and his family's medical lore. He went on journeys for research and to interview practitioners.

Both Li Shizhen's father and grandfather were doctors, and he grew up helping his father in his practice. Li's grandfather was a wondering country doctor who went around with a bag of herbs and medications and healed people. His father was a doctor and a scholar who had written several books. He wanted his son to enter the government by passing the Imperial Examination. Li studied for the exams and passed the country-level examination, but he was never able to pass the Imperial Examination.

When he was 27, he cured the son of a prince and was invited to be a doctor and official in that court. A few years later, he became an official at the Imperial Medical Institute in Beijing. During the years he spent there, he had access to rare and old medical texts. He also found that the available medical texts had inaccuracies and contradicted each other and that the medical knowledge of his time was not well defined. He wanted to compile correct information in a logical system of organization.

He wanted to survey all the available knowledge of his time and write the most accurate natural medical text ever written. He thought that the medical texts that were generally available were inaccurate and even had dangerous misinformation. He is thought of as a man who dedicated his life to his works.

To research for his book, he travelled extensively and gained first-hand experience with many herbs and regional folk remedies, and he consulted hundreds of books. He worked on the text for decades and tried to have it published both by a private printer and by the court.

His book was made so finely detailed and listed so many different herbs, medicinal minerals and medicinal animal parts that it was too big and heavy to be used by travelling doctors. The text was divided into many volumes. In his drive for accuracy and completeness, a lot of material is not useful for average practitioners, though it is useful for scholarly reference. It includes material on his understanding of geology, physics and other topics. It is also useful because he included a very long list of references. *Ben Cao Gang Mu* is considered the greatest scientific achievement of the Ming era.

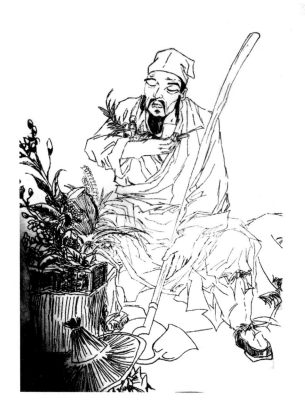

More reading

If you want to know more about TCM, please refer to the following links.

1.Hua Tuo | Chinese physician and surgeon | Britannica.com

https://www.britannica.com/biography/Hua-Tuo

2.Zhang Zhongjing—Sage of TCM

https://www.cchatty.com/article/Zhang-Zhongjing-Sage-of-TCM

3.Sun Simiao—King of Chinese Medicine

https://www.cchatty.com/article/Sun-Simiao-King-of-Chinese-Medicine

4.Li Shizhen: Scholar Worthy of Emulation

http://www.itmonline.org/arts/lishizhen.htm

Part Three
Stories in the History of TCM

This morning, one of my grandpa's patients came to express his gratitude. The patient told me he would have died without my grandpa's help. After he left, I said proudly to my grandpa, "You're the best, Grandpa!" But my grandpa shook his head and then he told me a story about Bian Que. The story goes like this.

1. King of Wei asking Bian Que

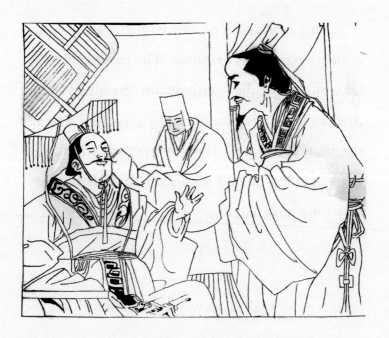

One day, the King of Wei called Bian Que to him and asked him, "I hear you have two brothers who are also physicians. Can you be honest and tell me who is the best physician among you three? "

Bian Que answered, "My eldest brother is the best. My second brother is better than me. Actually, I am just average." The king was surprised and said, "You are the one who is so famous that everyone knows you, while your brothers are not so famous. Why do you say they are better than you?" Bian Que answered, "My eldest brother believes in a lot of prevention. He looks for the source of illness and treats problems before people even feel anything. So, his patients don't even realize how much he has done for them, and they don't talk about him much. My second brother treats people at the first sign of a disease. They are having some symptoms, so he treats them before they get any worse. Because of this, people notice that he has helped them, and he has become well-known in our home town. As for me, people come to see me when they are already very sick. I use the strongest herbs, the most powerful acupuncture treatments. I even perform surgeries! Most of the time, I can't do anything to help them because they are already too ill. But sometimes I am able to save someone's life. That is the kind of thing people like to talk about, so I am the one who is the most famous." This is a very famous story in TCM history. So, I understood why my grandpa didn't think he was the best doctor: the best physician is the one who prevents his patients from becoming sick, not the one who tries to save them when they are already near death.

2. Bian Que Met King of Cai

Then my grandpa told me the second story which was also about Bian Que. In the kingdom of Qi, Bian Que came across the King of Cai, looked at him for a while and said, "You are ill. But it doesn't matter, since the sickness is yet skin deep. It is easy to cure." The king looked at him with his eyes partly closed and said, "Many thanks. But I need no treatment at all! I am very healthy and full of energy."

Bian Que shook his head and left without saying anything.

After his departure, the king said to his men, "That's the way a doctor shows his skills: treating healthy patients to cure non—illness."

Ten days later, the king met with Bian Que again and Bian Que told him once more, "Your Majesty, the sickness now has got into your muscles. You should not pay little attention to it. Please take some medicine."

The king wore a long face and ignored the advice.

Another ten days passed. Bian Que said to the king in earnest, "Really Your Majesty! The sickness is now already dwelling in your stomach and bowels. It will be mortal if you persist in objecting to a treatment in time!"

The king got annoyed and sniffed scornfully.

Thus a dozen more days had slipped by. One day hardly had Bian Que seen the king when he walked away. Quite puzzled, the king sent a man to find out the reason. When the man caught up with him, Bian Que replied, "It's curable when a disease doesn't develop to its fatal degree. But now, by refusing a treatment, His Majesty has allowed his illness into his marrow, a case that nobody can deal with successfully." Five days later, the king felt his body aching all over. At once he sent for Bian Que. But, Bian Que had anticipated this and he had long gone to Qin.

King of Cai died at last, filled with pain and regret.

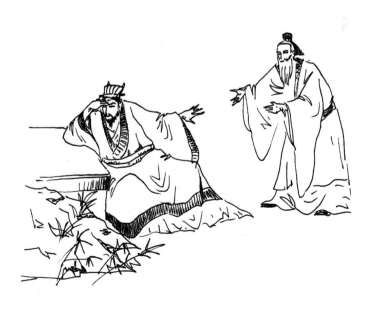

This story helped us to realize the importance of treating a disease at the outset.

Is Bian Que a brilliant doctor? Are you impressed with his exact diagnoses on the evolvement of disease through observing the complexion? I am! I became interested in him. Then I went on to find more information about him. Bian Que's surname is Qin and original given name is Yueren. He is a medical scientist living in the Warring States of China at the beginning of the 4th century B.C. As his medical knowledge was brilliant and he cured many diseases for common people, he was conferred the title of "Bian Que". It is the name of a legendary doctor who was a really good doctor in ancient time.

3. Hua Tuo and Crabs

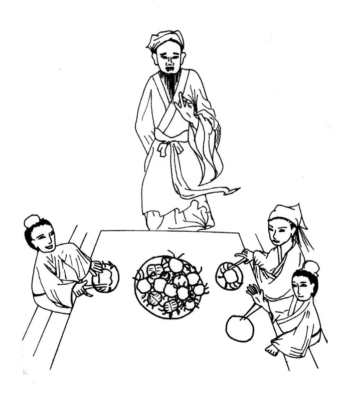

Many foods have similar effects like medicine. Overeating of some food may do harm to health. I'll tell you a story about Hua Tuo and crabs which I read in a TCM book about medicined diet. Hua Tuo and his apprentice Wu Pu were once in Suzhou, a delicate place in the south of China, which was famous for its beautiful scenery and delicious food. Hua Tuo liked delicious food very much.

Walking on the road, Hua Tuo was attracted by the smell of crabs. The owner of the restaurant came to greet him with a smile. Hua Tuo ordered two crabs. Wu Pu said, "Master, two crabs are so few. I myself can eat at least ten in a row." Hua Tuo smiled but said nothing, and then he took out of a book and began to read while waiting for the crabs.

Next to their table, three young men were enjoying crabs. The crab shells on their table almost piled up to the roof. Wu Pu envied that they could gorge themselves on delicious crabs and he intentionally pointed to them, indicating Hua Tuo ordered too few.

Hua Tuo was shocked to see so many crab shells. Then he looked at the faces of the three young men and squatted down to look at their bellies. Then he said to them, "Hey, young men! Crabs are cold in property. It's easy to get sick if you eat too much. You've already eaten enough. It's dangerous to eat more."

The three young men were enjoying themselves, and they were very unhappy to hear Hua Tuo's words. One of them was called Fan, who was a warrior and famous for his strong and healthy body.

"Old man, it's none of your business. I am rich and can afford as much as I want!" said Fan.

Wu Pu noticed other two young men were

looking at them aggressively, and then he stopped Hua Tuo. Hua Tuo said to Wu Pu, "I have to stop them. Look at their complexion! They had too many crabs but they didn't know. They will get sick soon if they don't stop."

The owner of the restaurant heard this and walked to Hua Tuo, "Mind yourself! Don't disturb my business!" He whispered to Hua Tuo in a very unfriendly voice.

Sighing, Hua Tuo shook his head.

Not long after that, a cry of anguish burst from the lips of the three young men who were clutching their stomach. Fan shouted at the boss, "your crabs are poisonous! "

The boss was too nervous to argue. Hua Tuo helped the boss out and said, "It is not that the crabs are poisonous, but you are sick. I've told you crabs are delicious but they are cold in property. When you eat too much, your stomach is harmed and you get sick."

The three young men cried with pain. Fan begged, "Help! Please help us! It kills. I'll give you money as much as you ask." "I don't need your money," Hua Tuo smiled, "I need you to remember food has properties. Don't indulge!" Fan nodded his head. "Sure, I won't any more."

Hua Tuo said to Wu Pu, "Let's find the medicine."Wu Pu followed him to the vegetable garden next to the restaurant and gathered some purple leaves. Hua Tuo asked the boss for some ginger. He put the purple leaves and ginger in a pot and boiled them with some water. The three young men took the water and they felt much better. About two hours later, they were fine and didn't feel uncomfortable any more.

Ashamedly, Fan apologized to Hua Tuo, "I'm sorry. Thank you for saving us. But what are the leaves?" Hua Tuo explained, "This is a good thing. It is very effective for the discomfort caused by eating too many crabs and shrimps. The leaves can also help to get rid of symptoms of cold. Because it is purple and it is good for the stomach, so I name it Purple Su."

Wu Pu was surprised and asked, "Master, I've never read it in any book. How could you know its functions?" Hua Tuo said, "One day, by a river, I saw an otter with a swollen belly because of eating too much. It seemed that he didn't feel well and was searching for something anxiously. When it found purple perilla, it chewed the leaves. After a while, it was all right. Then I knew the purple leaves could heal indigestion."

After hearing the words, they admired Hua Tuo more.

Bian Que and Hua Tuo found out the patients' problems by observing their complexion. TCM doctors not only treat patients by observing but by investigating their daily routine and lifestyle. The following story is about Sun Simiao, the famous physician I've introduced to you, who cured a weird illness by changing patients' eating habits.

4. Sun Simiao Curing Weird Disease

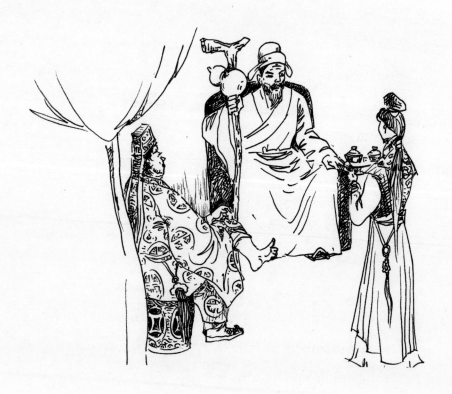

According to legend, in the Tang dynasty, some people suffered from a strange disease. They continued to have fatigue and weakness. Their legs were heavy and the muscles were sore. They suffered from swollen ankles and burning foot. Some complained they felt stings on the feet and sometimes they felt as if ants were crawling on their feet. They didn't have a good appetite. Many people were not found better after medical treatment.

At that time, a governor also suffered from the disease, so he invited the famous doctor Sun Simiao to his home. At first, Sun Simiao didn't know how to treat it. But he asked to stay there for several days, and then he found that all servants there were healthy only the governor and his family members had the disease. Sun Simiao talked to a butler and the butler told him the rice the governor's family had was all carefully ground and sieved before making into staple food. Later, he went to other patients' houses to investigate. He found all the patients were wealthy people, especially some high officials and noble lords. And all of them only had elaborately processed grains. The poor and their servants who had whole grains for meals were healthy. Sun Simiao concluded these rich people's fine staple food was the main cause of their illness.

Therefore he asked these families to change the original use of refined rice noodles to coarse rice noodles as a staple food. Grain bran was boiled and they were also asked to drink large amounts of bran water instead of tea. A month later, all the rich patients recovered from the weird disease.

Sun Simiao was really awesome, do you think so? The weird disease is actually called beriberi. It's mainly caused by a lack of vitamin B in food. Vitamin B is mainly found in the outer skin and germ of grains such as rice, millet, wheat, barley, buckwheat, oat, etc. Therefore, we do not recommend daily consumption of overly fine rice noodles. Once suffering from beriberi, people with mild disease can eat more of the above mentioned food. As for those serious symptoms, patients need medical treatment.

There are a great many stories in the history of TCM, which help us to understand TCM better. If you want to know more about TCM, please refer to the following links.

More reading

1.Bian Que—Ancestor of TCM

https://www.cchatty.com/article/Bian–
Que–Ancestor–of–TCM

2.Fact Versus Myth: Traditional Chinese
Medicine

https://www.borgenmagazine.com/fact–
versus–myth–traditional–chinese–medicine/

Part Four

Knowing Chinese Herbal Medicine

1. Story of Shennong

Have you heard about Shennong? The story of "Shennong tasting hundreds of herbs" is a famous legend since ancient China. Then I will tell you the story.

In ancient time, people lived on hunting. However, because of poor tools, the animals people caught were not enough to eat. Legend had it that there was a man named Shennong, a famous leader of an ancient tribe, who taught people to cultivate and grow crops. He also led his people to make all kinds of farm implements and build water conservancy. In this way, people were able to survive.

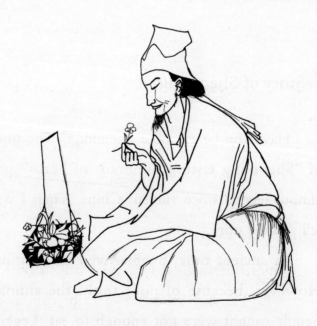

However, due to horrible national environment and bad living conditions, many people suffered from various diseases, and sometimes they might eat some poisonous plants as they knew very little of different plants. It seemed that people usually had no choice but to wait for their death. Therefore, Shennong who cared about his people made up his mind to help them. So whenever he came across some plants that he didn't know, he would observe their appearance, taste them himself, and record his feelings and the effects of the plants. In this way, he was able to find out which plants were safe and edible, and even could cure people's diseases, and which plants were harmful to people's health.

Sometimes, he would even run the risk of losing his life. Legend had it that one day he was poisoned seriously when tasting some strange plants. Feeling dizzy, he had to rest against a big tree, and his life was in danger. Suddenly, he smelt some fresh fragrance in the breeze, and found some green leaves falling slowly from the tree. He picked up a leaf and chewed it. After few seconds, he felt refreshed and energetic again. He named this plant "Cha", which is known as tea later. Even though he came across millions of dangers and difficulties, he never gave up his target of helping his people to find out herbs to cure their diseases.

It is often believed that one day when he tasted a special herb named gelsemium elegan or "duan chang cao" in Chinese, he was poisoned seriously. The poison in this herb was so terrible that he wasn't able to eat tea leaves to detoxify it, and thus he unfortunately died.

Shennong has made much contribution to the development of Chinese agriculture and medicine in ancient China. Thanks to his efforts, people in that time were able to have enough food to survive, and many people who got diseases or poisoned were saved from death. Even today, he is still memorized and respected by many Chinese people.

2. Medicine? Food? Both!

Sometimes I don't like some vegetables such as carrots and celeries, and my grandpa always tells me not to be a picky eater. He tells me that a balanced diet is very important for our bodies and many foods actually have similar effects like medicine. I asked why and he explained in this way.

Chinese medicine and food are closely related according to traditional Chinese medical theories. Chinese medicine mainly comes from various herbs, animals and minerals, while the food that people have every day also comes from the same things in nature. It can be said that Chinese medicine and food have the same origins. And a lot of herbs, animals and some minerals can be taken both as medicine and food since they can not only feed people but also have curative effects on certain diseases. Like Chinese medicine, each food also has its special functions. Therefore, for thousands of years, TCM emphasized a balanced diet and adjustment of diet according to the changing of physical condition of individuals.

How wonderful Chinese medicine is! Do you believe that many foods in our kitchen and on our dining tables actually have curative effects just like medicine? And many of these foods are even often used by traditional Chinese doctors to treat their patients. In our daily life, if properly used, they can be of great benefit to our health. The following are two stories that I once experienced:

"The ice-cream event"
—ginger, mung beans and Chinese yam

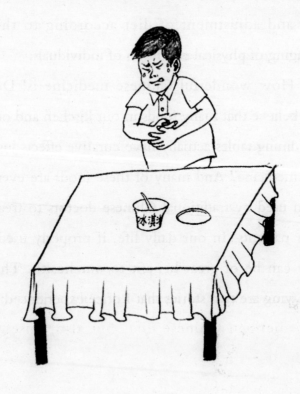

In summer when it's extremely hot, I am always eager to have something cold even though my grandpa often says it's not good for my health. But who can resist the temptation of cold drinks and ice-cream on a hot summer day? One day I played soccer with my friends, and when I got home I felt so hot that I had some cold coke and then much ice-cream. Therefore at night I had a stomachache. After knowing what happened to me, my grandpa went to the kitchen and twenty minutes later, he came out with a bowl of strange soup. He told me to drink this dark red soup. I will never forget its special taste—spicy and sweet. But strangely, after drinking it, I did feel much better. Grandpa said this soup was made of ginger and brown sugar. Ginger is not only a common ingredient in Chinese diet, but also a useful medicine as it can be refreshing and promote people's appetite. Besides, when people get cold, ginger soup will do them good because ginger can dispel the coldness in the human body.

After that, Grandpa told me to stop having too much ice-cream and asked me to drink some green soup he specially made for me when the weather was hot. The soup was light green, with a little bit bitter and sweet taste. I wondered why Grandpa asked me to drink this strange soup, but amazingly, I found I did feel cooler after drinking it in the hot summer days. Grandpa told me the soup was made of mung beans. He explained to me that mung beans were highly praised by Li Shizhen as "a good grain that benefits mankind" because mung beans with a sweet but cold property could help people clear heat in the body. Therefore, mung bean soup which can help people reduce summer heat is one of the most popular drinks in summer for Chinese people.

Besides, the pillows stuffed with mung bean seed coat can improve eyesight, refresh the mind and reduce headache. Why don't you also try some mung bean soup when it's hot in summer?

On one weekend after the ice-cream event, I accompanied my mother to buy some vegetables in the supermarket. In the supermarket, we bought several different kinds of vegetables, and I noticed my mother also bought something strange. They are long, thin, brown sticks with muds and lots of hairs on the outside. Wow, they are ugly, and they must taste terrible, I thought secretly. In the evening, when my mother steamed some of this strange and ugly vegetable, and asked me to have some, I was amazed by its good taste. It tasted really good especially when being taken with some sugar. My mother told me she had bought this vegetable for me. I asked why. She said this special vegetable was Chinese yam, a very common vegetable in Chinese diet. It can be steamed, boiled in porridge, stir fried, or made into various desserts. However, it is not only tasteful but also beneficial for people's health. Many traditional Chinese doctors consider it as one of the most important medicines to make people stronger since it is good for our stomach and it's very nutritious. Therefore, my mother wanted to help me improve my stomach conditions. So why don't you also try some of Chinese yam when you have some stomach problems? Though it benefits a lot, you cannot have too much of it, as having too much of it may result in abdominal distention.

"An unforgettable Spring Festival"
—hawthorn fruit, pear, wild chrysanthemum flower and honeysuckle flower

What festival do you like best? Christmas is the most important festival in many western countries. However, in China, the most important festival is Spring Festival, or Chinese New Year. Almost all the children love it because we can enjoy a lot of delicious food, play firecrackers, put on new clothes, and receive lucky money. I am no exception. Each year long before Spring Festival, I always look forward to this holiday with eager expectancy because I can have a wonderful time during the Spring Festival. I still remember an interesting story that happened during this year's Spring Festival.

On the Eve of Spring Festival, we used to have a family reunion dinner prepared by my grandparents at home. But this year, my parents decided that we would have the dinner in a fancy restaurant so that my grandparents wouldn't be tired preparing for the dinner. That night, we had a wonderful time. Unfortunately, I had too much food and I felt uncomfortable in my stomach. Grandpa said what I had was indigestion and I needn't take any medicine. Instead, he asked me to take some hawthorn fruits. Hawthorn fruits? Could the red, lovely round fruits cure my problem? I highly doubted it, but I still took his advice and had some. Luckily, the second day, I found myself recovered. I wondered why this fruit was able to deal with my indigestion and asked Grandpa for the answer. He said hawthorn fruits could promote gastric acid secretion and thus help people increase appetite and deal with indigestion. When I asked more hawthorn fruits, my grandpa said no. He told me having too much of it might result in acid reflux. If you don't like its sour taste, there are also some delicious food made of hawthorn fruit such as haw jelly, haw slices and haw rolls. I'm sure you will enjoy them.

During this Spring Festival holiday, I went to play firecrackers with my friends. We had such a wonderful time that I forgot the time and got home too late. Since it was really cold that day, next morning I felt a little headache and had a runny nose.

"Dongdong, I think you've got a cold because of cold wind," said Grandpa after observing my symptoms.

"Cold? Then I think I can take some ginger soup." I still remember Grandpa has told me the functions of ginger.

"Yes, you are clever. But this time we also need something else besides ginger," Grandpa answered mysteriously.

"What can we try this time?" I was really curious about what he mentioned.

Then he went to the kitchen and came out with some green vegetables.

"This!" he said.

I noticed what in his hand was some Chinese onions. "Mom cooks dishes with them every day. How can they treat colds?" I blurted out.

"Don't look down upon them. Chinese onion and ginger can stimulate secretion of sweat, so they can help you with your cold. We just need to cut the white root parts of Chinese onions, and boil them together with some ginger and brown sugar. You must feel much better after drinking the soup." Grandpa explained patiently while he was busy preparing for my soup.

As expected, I was much better after I drank this special soup.

Several days later, I still had a sore throat and coughed a lot. This time, I went to ask Grandpa for advice because I was sure he must have some good ideas. He said, "You can eat some pears. Or you can also cook pear soup with rock sugar. This time can you cook it by yourself?"

"That sounds yummy. I like pears. But how can I cook this soup?"

"It's very easy. Cut the pears into small pieces, and boil them together with rock sugar for half an hour. Drink the soup twice a day, and three days later you can feel better."

Then I did what Grandpa told me. How sweet the soup was! I loved it. Several days later, I did feel much better.

But one day I came across Grandma Li, a neighbor living next door. I greeted her politely, "Good morning Grandma Li." She smiled and nodded to me, and then coughed.

Thinking she might also have got a cold, I told her, "Grandma Li, do you have a sore throat and cough a lot? My grandpa has taught me a good prescription, pear soup. It's sweet and I love it. Why not try some?"

She smiled and answered, "Thank you, Dongdong. But I have diabetes, and I dare not take anything sweet."

"Oh, I'm sorry to hear that. Then I will go home and ask my grandpa what you can do to cure your sore throat."

"Thank you. You are such a warm-hearted boy." Grandma Li said to me.

After I got home, I told my grandpa about

Grandma Li, and then asked, "Grandpa, what can she do if she can't drink pear soup?"

"People with diabetes can have pear soup, but they can't have too much. Still I will tell you two flowers which are good for throat problems." He said.

"Flowers?" I was puzzled.

Can flowers cure diseases? That's unbelievable.

"Yes," he answered. "They are wild chrysanthemum flower and honeysuckle flower. These two flowers both have the cold property, and they not only can help people with throat problems but also have other effects. For example, wild chrysanthemum flower is also helpful for people with coronary heart disease and high blood pressure. It is also good for our eyesight. Honeysuckle flower can help cure inflammation and has heat—clearing and detoxifying effect. So it's one of the main ingredients of herbal tea."

Thanks to Grandpa, I can learn a lot of medical knowledge about the amazing foods and use them to cure myself and help other people. Besides the foods I mentioned above, what other foods do you know that have curative effects on various diseases? Go to your kitchen and you can find more answers. I hope you can share your own stories with me and of course with your friends.

More reading

If you want to know more about TCM, please refer to the following links.

1. The Benefits of Traditional Chinese Medicine—Dr. Axe

https://draxe.com/traditional−chinese−medicine/

2. An Introduction to Chinese Herbs

http://www.itmonline.org/arts/herbintro.htm

3.Food As Medicine: TCM−Inspired Healthy Eating Principles with Action Guide, Worksheet, and 10−Week Meal Plan to Restore Health, Beauty, and Mind

https://www.amazon.com/Food−Medicine−Traditional−Medicine−Inspired−Principles/dp/150787670X

Part Five

Health Preservation in TCM

Hi, everyone! In this part, I'll talk about health preservation. Health preservation used to be a common topic for senior citizens in China, however, modern young people are also paying attention to it.

1. The Understanding of Health in TCM

How will you define health if you're asked to? You might answer health means I have a strong body and I'm free from illness. Yes, strong body and no illness mean health. But the young who have strong bodies do have a range of uncomfortable symptoms but without obvious illnesses. According to TCM, they are not healthy since health has three aspects in TCM. Firstly, one's physical body functions well with a symbol of smooth operation of qi and blood. Secondly, a healthy person must have normal and sound mental activities. Finally, a person can adapt himself/herself to outside environment and his/her physical condition. In a word, health in TCM includes the harmony between qi and blood, body and mentality, nature and human.

A Butcher Dismembering an Ox

You may have found that health preservation in TCM emphasizes much on the importance of following nature. In TCM the core of health preservation is conforming to nature. I'll tell you a

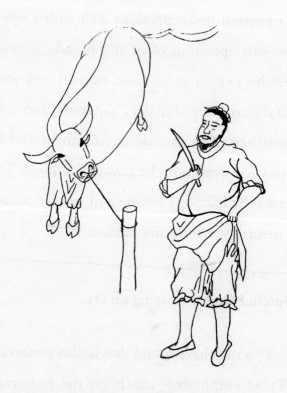

story titled *A Butcher Dismembering an Ox*.

One day a butcher was cutting up an ox. He was so skillful that it seemed that every part his hand reached fell apart without any of his efforts. King Wenhui was so surprised to see this. He asked the butcher, "How could you be so perfect in doing this?" The butcher answered, "Natural openings exist between the ox's muscles, and crevices in its joints. I don't see the ox with my eyes. It is in my mind. I just lead my knife into the openings and through the crevices." Hearing his words, King Wenhui responded, "I figure out the way of nurturing life, which is to follow the nature." When we live our life by following nature, we are sure to be healthy. For example, when the sun rises, we get up and begin to work. We go to bed when the sun sets. It actually means we should have a regular rhythm of work and rest.

2. Common Ways to Preserve Health

Is it possible for you to live over 100 years old? Do you know the ways to preserve your health? Under the guidance of TCM theories, Chinese people have always been emphasizing health preservation and longevity. The activities of health preservation run through the whole of one's life, from birth, growth, aging to death. By various methods, health preservation helps to enhance the health and increase longevity. Common methods include mental preservation, diet adjusting, body building, climate adaptation and etc. In the following let me introduce you one by one.

2.1 Mental preservation

TMC believes human spiritual activities directly influence one's physical health. Improper mental activities may result in disfunction of human body and imbalance between qi and blood. A well-known Chinese story proves this vividly. There was once a man named Fan Jin in the Qing dynasty. He made every effort to pass the civil exam. He failed again and again. One day he was in the depth of despair when he got the news that he had finally passed it. The sudden excitement damaged his mentality, and he ecstatically ran to tell everyone he knew. He lost his shoe without knowing. He fell down the gutter but he was unaware of it. He was mad. In the end his father-in-law to whom he was always frightened slapped him on the face and helped him regain reason. This story shows sudden extreme ecstasy does harm to one's health. To keep healthy, one needs to nourish his/her mental activities. In TCM a good health preserver always keeps optimistic, worries little, desires little and maintains a good mentality to everything in his life.

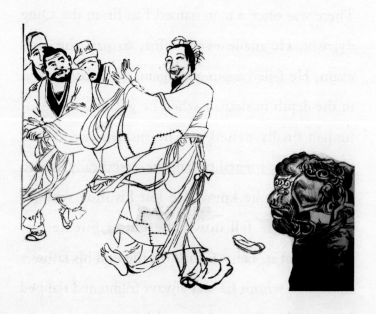

2.2 Diet adjusting

TCM believes the refined materials in food are the source of human energy. Different kinds of food have different kinds of functions and effects. Chinese people generally believe some common food has specific effects on health preservation. For example, white radish can moisten lungs and black beans tonify kidneys. A balanced diet helps to nourish your life and guarantee your health. In modern society, many people are persisting bad eating habits all year around. Junk food and fried food taste well, but too much of them brings risks to human health. Chinese people generally believe diseases result from the food you take from your mouth. To be healthy, people need to pay much attention to the quality of food. In TCM it is believed that each kind of food has its own property. For example, the property of mung beans is coldness. It helps to clear away heat and toxic material. In midsummer, most Chinese people cannot do without a bowl of mung beans soup.

TCM believes different food also protects or nourishes different parts of human body. Spinach protects brain. Seaweed is good for hair. Tomatoes benefit lungs and etc. If you don't feel well, or you find some parts of your body need improvement, you can eat the corresponding food. Stick to it consistently, your situation will gradually improve. You may find all food I mention is natural. We Chinese don't prefer processed food. Naturalness is the key factor in healthy diet.

Chinese people put much emphasis on grains which are regarded as the source of our life. An idiom "a bumper grain harvest" in Chinese symbolizes happiness. For thousands of years, our ancestors thrived on grains that inspired generations to multiply. These humble grains carry countless lives and have extraordinary health care value. In my family, millet congee is indispensable on our table. My mother often cooks millet with longans, which is the perfect tonic for the old and the sick because it can nourish blood, soothe nerves and improve intelligence. All you need to remember is to eat more grains. But don't eat grains which are refined too much.

2.3 Water drinking

Nobody can deny the importance of water. When it comes to drinking water, everyone feels it is simple, but do you know how to drink water properly? When do you need to drink? What water is the best for health preservation?

Some people drink two or three cups of

water in a row and then do not drink water for four or five hours. Or they do not drink during the day but drink water at night. This is very bad for the body. In TCM, water is regarded as the lifeblood. When drinking water, you need to bear the following principles in mind:

Firstly, drink a little but for several times. Drinking too much or too little at a time is not good for health. The commonly accepted method in TCM is to drink a glass of water (about 200 ~ 250 milliliters) at a time.

Secondly, drink water regularly. Some people do not form the habit of drinking water regularly. Only when they feel thirsty do they realize it is time to have some water. When you are thirsty, in fact, your body is warning you about the lack of water. You need to have enough water immediately. It is better to have water regularly instead of waiting till you feel thirsty.

Thirdly, don't drink too fast. Drinking water too fast may swallow air together leading to hiccup or flatulence. Some may drink a lot of water at one time, especially after exhausting exercises. The proper way to drink water after tough exercise is to moisten your mouth and throat first, then drink a little water slowly. Wait for a moment then drink a little more. Your body needs time to calm and restore. Follow the rhythm of your body, and you'll keep healthy.

2.4 Tea drinking

You may know Chinese people like drinking tea. Drinking tea is regarded as a way to preserve health, and it can also cure various diseases, because tea has elements good to health, which has been proven by modern medicine. It helps to satisfy both the need of body and mind. The reason why Chinese people like to drink tea is that they know that drinking tea not only satisfies physical need, more importantly, it helps to keep healthy. Drinking tea is said to be a science. TCM believe people need to choose different types of tea based on their constitution. A person, with a constitution of yang deficiency characterized by cold limbs, pale complexion, and easy to catch a cold, shouldn't drink green tea. It is suggested that they drink more black tea.

Do you like drinking tea? What's your favorite tea? Does it fit your constitution? If you are not sure, consult a TCM doctor.

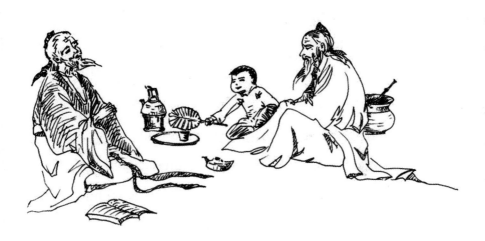

2.5 Qigong

Qigong is one of the most important ways in health preservation. In many Chinese martial arts novels, qigong is described as something that can help people walk on walls and fly over the roofs. It is actually not that magical, but it does do good to health. It is the way to regulate or balance qi in your body and helps to preserve both physical and mental health. TCM believes physical diseases are partially caused by mental problems including emotional stress. Therefore to preserve health, cultivating one's inner tranquility is the first and foremost thing people need to do. Many Chinese people practice qigong to get a healthier body and more balanced mind. Qigong helps to feel the energy in your body, which allows you to know the situation of your thoughts and emotions.

Do you want to learn to practice qigong to

become a qigong master? You may think you need a dense forest to practice it. Without the hazy forest, can we practice qigong? Sure! We can. To tell you the truth, it's not easy to be a qigong master, but it's easy to practice qigong. Qigong, a general term, includes different styles. Here, I can teach you one named Baduanjin qigong. My grandfather practices it every morning. Baduanjin qigong includes eight moves. It is easy to learn and you can practice it at almost any place you like. There are eight sections. You may refer to the following drawing.

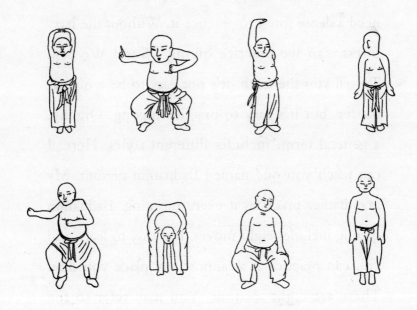

Baduanjin Qigong

The sequence is not fixed. You may pick one or two of them to practice.

The name of each exercise is listed as follows:

1. Palms raised to heaven

2. Drawing the bow

3. Separating heaven and earth

4. The wise owl gazes backward

5. Punching with angry eyes

6. Press the earth, touch the sky

7. Shake the head & swing tail

8. Lifting up the heels

Many videos about Baduanjin qigong exist in the Internet. If you are really interested in it, you may search the key words "Baduanjin" in your Internet search engine.

2.6 Tai Ji

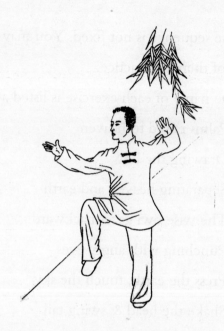

Tai Ji is a centuries–old mind and body practice. It involves gentle, dance–like body movements with mental focus, breathing, and relaxation. Although it was originally regarded as a martial art, it is also practiced to achieve greater longevity.

118

Some describe Tai Ji as "meditation in motion", but more call it "medication in motion". More and more evidence shows that it has value in treating or preventing many health problems. And you can get started even if you aren't in top shape or the best of health. You may also find Tai Ji appealing because it's inexpensive and requires no special equipment. You can do Tai Ji anywhere, including indoors or outdoors. And you can do it alone or in a group class. Easy as it is to get started, you still need to check with your doctor if you have a limiting medical condition. Given its excellent safety record, chances are that you'll be encouraged to try it.

3. Self-healthcare Tuina Therapy

Besides the above ways you may adopt in your life, self−healthcare Tuina is also a very important way in health preservation. In ancient times, it is named "daoyin (导引)" in Chinese. Let me show you several simple ones to help you to relieve your fatigue or to improve your sleep.

3.1 Techniques to relieve fatigue

When you feel tired, what do you need to do? Of course, you need to take a rest. You can also alleviate your tiredness in the following ways.

Soothing heart and calming mind

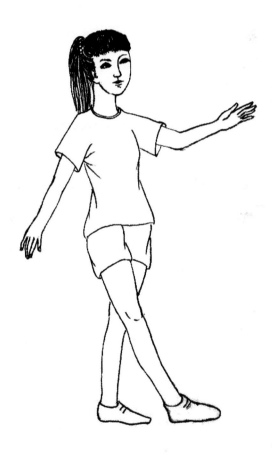

First you take a position of standing, your feet with shoulder width apart. Relax yourself with your hands stretched naturally. Rotate your waist, your arms and your elbows sway with your body. When your waist turns to the left, you pat your left chest with your right palm in your front. Meanwhile, your left hand moves to your back, and pat your back on the right with your left hand back. Then do the same as your waist turns to your right. If you do this for the first time, pat gently. If you don't feel uncomfortable, you may pat harder next time. Do this for 36 times as one round.

Stretching your chest and waist

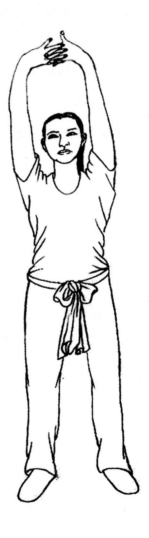

Take a standing position. Cross your figures with palms upward and extend your arms upwards to the highest you can reach. Take a deep breath as you move your back backwards. Then bend your body forward to let your palms reach the ground while taking the breath out. Remember, don't bend your knee joints and stand firmly during the whole process. Repeat the movement 9 times.

3.2 Techniques to improve sleep

Is your sleep sound or shallow? Do you have difficulty in falling asleep? Can you have enough sleep every night? TCM believes sleep is the best way to recover and preserve health. For many people, it's not easy to enjoy a sound, sweet sleep due to many factors. Here is an easy way that might not be magical but it does help for some people.

Sedating mind and benefiting sleep

First you need to regulate your breath. You may lie on your back or just sit quietly. Take a deep and slow breath, hold it for one second, and try to exhale as much as possible. Repeat for 36 times. After regulating your breath, you can use the thumb of your right hand to press the left acupoint called Zusanli forcefully for 60 seconds. Then do the same on the opposite side.

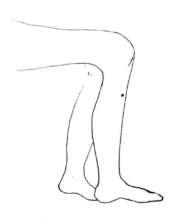

Applying "pushing" on your head and face

Take a sitting position. Put your palms on your forehead and your fingers on your head, then push upwards, keep pushing till your palms slide down the back of your head. Stop until your palms reach the side of your neck. Repeat it for 9 times.

Sure, there are more acupoints you need to press. Forgive me! I can't explain all of them one by one as they are really complicated. I hope you can improve your sleep quality by regulating breath and pressing Zusanli.

There are tons of methods in self–healthcare Tuina therapy. You may have found one of the benefits is that you can practice them by yourself.

After I've introduced you so many ways to preserve health, do you have confidence to live more than 100 years? I hope you can. But to tell you the truth, the fulfillment of health longevity not only depends on the knowledge of the methods of health preservation, but also on the proper application of these methods to daily life and making it one part of life. So, don't be lazy. Move! Move now! Enjoy your longevity in the future!

More reading

If you want to know more about TCM, please refer to the following links.

1. Health Preservation and TCM

https://confuciusmag.com/health-preservation-chinese-medicine

2. Preservation of Mental Health

https://www.centarsrce.org/en/ocuvanje_mentalnog_zdravlja.php

3. Food Therapy and Medical Diet Therapy of TCM

https://www.sciencedirect.com/science/article/pii/S2352939317300829

4. Eight Steps to Healthy Living

http://www.baduanjin.com/english/ba-duan-jin/

Part Six

The Internationalization of TCM

1. The Law of the People's Republic of China on TCM

The Chinese government has granted greater importance to the development of TCM, and made a series of major policy decisions and adopted a number of plans in this regard. In 2014, the State Council Information Office of China issued its first white paper on the development of TCM, detailing policies and measures on TCM development and highlighting its unique value in the new era. In 2016, State Administration of TCM issued the "Thirteenth Five–year Plan" for Cultural Construction of TCM, promoting the further development of TCM in China. The State Council issued the Outline of the Strategic Plan on the Development of TCM (2016—2030) in 2016, which made TCM development a national strategy.

As an old Chinese saying goes, "Nothing can be accomplished without rules." More than 30 years ago, a group of well–known experts made many suggestions for the rapid development of TCM rules. The rules not only confirmed the basic responsibilities and rights of every TCM doctor, but also regulated the management procedures of hospitals. The Law of the People's Republic of China on TCM was issued on December 25, 2016 and it is the first national law on TCM. It was formulated to safeguard and promote TCM development and protect people's health. The Law was formally implemented on July 1, 2017, providing a sounder policy environment and legal basis for TCM development. It has become a symbol of the development of TCM as a national strategy. TCM has also opened a new phase of comprehensive development. It is also the first comprehensive and systematic law to embody the uniqueness of TCM in China. All the decisions and plans have mapped out a grand blueprint for the development of TCM in a new era.

2. TCM and the Nobel Prize

Do you know Tu Youyou who won the 2011 Lasker Award in Clinical Medicine and the 2015 Nobel Prize in Physiology or Medicine? She is a researcher of China Academy of Chinese Medical Sciences who drew inspiration from *Zhou Hou Bei Ji Fang* (《肘后备急方》*A handbook of Prescriptons for Emergencies*) and other traditional Chinese literature for the discovery of qinghaosu (artemisinin), an anti–alaria drug.

Malaria is an acute infectious disease, which infects more than 300 million people in more than 100 countries. In 1969, Tu Youyou was an intern researcher at Chinese Academy of TCM. She read a large number of traditional medicine classics, consulted the old Chinese medicine experts and collected more than 2,000 prescriptions. After obtaining the sample, Tu herself was the first to test the drug in person. After successful trials, a series of safety tests and the first clinical trial were conducted. Thanks to her discovery, 200 million people were saved. Tu was the first Chinese to win the Nobel Prize for natural science. It is also the highest award TCM has achieved.

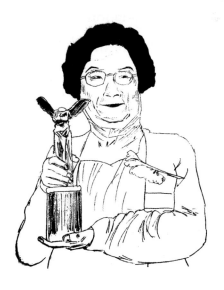

3. New progress in TCM culture

In China, efforts have been reinforced to promote public awareness in TCM healthcare. The campaign of TCM Across China initiated in 2007 by some 20 government bodies including the National Administration of TCM (NATCM) aims to increase public understanding of TCM and promote its wider use in the community. Public talks have been organized through media and TCM education bases, popularizing basic knowledge and skills of TCM healthcare and prevention and treatment of illnesses. In this way, public awareness and ability to practice TCM healthcare has been enhanced and general public health has improved. The results of the survey on health culture literacy of TCM in 2016 released by NATCM show that in 2016, the popularization rate of TCM knowledge in China was 91.86%, and the level of health culture literacy of Chinese citizens was 12.85%.

The Chinese government treasures and protects the cultural value of TCM. With the support of our country, one hundred and thirty TCM elements have been incorporated into the Representative List of National Intangible Cultural Heritage. In 2010 Chinese acupuncture was listed in the UNESCO Human Intangible Cultural Heritage Representative List. In 2010 TCM acupuncture and moxibustion was included in the Representative List of the Intangible Cultural Heritage of Humanity by UNESCO. In 2011 the *Huang Di Nei Jing* (*Yellow Emperor's Inner Canon*) and *Ben Cao Gang Mu* was listed in the Memory of the World Register. A number of Chinese medicine standards have been formulated and cooperation bases have been established. TCM is on the road of being internationalized.

Do you want to learn TCM? If you're in China, you can come to TCM universities or colleges. In China there are more than 20 universities with lots of excellent TCM teachers and doctors. There are 10 TCM academicians, 90 masters of TCM and 100 famous national TCM doctors in China. They are all representatives of excellent TCM practitioners.

4. TCM walks to the world

TCM was born in China, and it has also absorbed the essence of other civilizations, and gradually spread throughout the world. At present, Chinese medicine has been put in use in 183 countries and regions, passed to the people of the world. Cooperative protocols have been signed on Chinese medicine between 86 countries and China. China has founded 17 TCM centres abroad.

What's more, many foreigners are very interested in TCM acupuncture, massage and herbal medicine, and some countries have even set up Confucius Institutes to teach TCM. Up to December 31, 2017, there are 525 Confucius

Institutes in 138 countries and regions, including 118 in 33 countries and regions of Asia, 54 in 39 countries of Africa, 173 in 41 countries of Europe, 161 in 21 countries of America and 19 in 4 countries of Oceania.

Among them, you may get more information about TCM in the following places: Chinese Medicine Confucius Institute at RMIT University, the London Confucius Institute for TCM at London South Bank University, Chinese Medicine Confucius Institute at Hyogo College of Medicine, Confucius Classroom at Kobe Toyo Medical School and Confucius Institute for TCM at Huachiew Chalermprakiet University.

What's more, some countries regularly invite teachers from China to teach TCM courses. In order to learn more about Chinese medicine, many foreigners come to China and find Chinese medicine experts to learn from. Foreigners who have learned Chinese medicine will say excitedly, "The treatment of diseases in Chinese medicine is amazing. A small silver needle can cure so many diseases. If not to learn personally, it is really difficult to believe it!"

TCM is a key component in exchanges between China and the rest of the world in improving the well-being of humanity, and developing a community of shared future. There are both opportunities and challenges for TCM nowadays. As a Chinese, I am proud to introduce it to you. I hope you can have a chance to know it better and to experience it by yourself. You'll find it is really interesting.

More reading

If you want to know more about TCM, please refer to the following links.

1. Confucius Institute at LSBU

https://lsbu−confucius.london/

2. Mr. Sohei Shinka: A Man Devoted to the Introduction of TCM

https://confuciusmag.com/sohei−shinka−traditional−chinese−medicine